Advancing Conversations: Aubrey de Grey

T0154589

Advancing Conversations: Aubrey de Grey

Douglas Lain

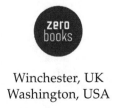

Winchester, UK
Washington, USA

First published by Zero Books, 2016
Zero Books is an imprint of John Hunt Publishing Ltd., Laurel House, Station Approach,
Alresford, Hants, SO24 9JH, UK
office1@jhpbooks.net
www.johnhuntpublishing.com
www.zero-books.net

For distributor details and how to order please visit the 'Ordering' section on our website.

Text copyright: Douglas Lain 2015

ISBN: 978 1 78535 396 3
Library of Congress Control Number: 2015960676

A CIP catalogue record for this book is available from the British Library.

Design: Lee Nash

Printed and bound by CPI Group (UK) Ltd, Croydon, CR0 4YY, UK

We operate a distinctive and ethical publishing philosophy in all
areas of our business, from our global network of authors to
production and worldwide distribution.

CONTENTS

Preface

Aubrey de Grey is the Chief Science Officer of SENS Research Foundation, an organization dedicated to a damage-repair model designed to combat the diseases of old age by fixing or undoing the damage the body does to itself simply by being alive. That title, "Chief Science Officer," might sound a bit science-fictional, especially in the context of life extension, but de Grey is adamant that his approach to gerontology is anything but science fiction. As improbable as his claims sound – he suggests that medical science is on the cusp of developing technologies that will, through progressive improvements that stay one step ahead of the problem, extend the average human life into four digits – de Grey insists that the science behind his organization is solid. SENS stands for Strategies for Engineered Negligible Senescence, and the strategy for rejuvenating aging human bodies involves going after seven types of molecular and cellular damage caused by normal metabolic functioning. The full list of damage is as follows: cell loss, cancerous cells, mitochondrial mutations, death-resistant cells, extracellular matrix stiffening, extracellular aggregates, and intracellular aggregates. The remedies for these seven different types of damage include the use of Stem cells, the removal of telomere-lengthening machinery, targeted ablation, and novel lysosomal hydrolases and more. What is unique about the SENS approach is that, rather than attempting to slow down the creation of damage or merely address the various diseases that result from the damage once it becomes intolerably abundant, de Grey and his team propose to intervene with the aim of repair and maintenance of that damage. On the SENS Research site the organization claims, "The specific metabolic processes that are ultimately responsible for causing all of this damage are still only partially understood. The good news is that we don't need to answer the many open questions about the causes of structural decay in order to develop effective therapies to reverse it. No matter what caused a given unit of damage in the first place, the same regenerative therapeutics can be used to repair it. In other words, it doesn't matter how a given microscopic lesion occurred, if we apply rejuvenation biotechnologies that restore the machinery of life to proper working order. "Aubrey de Grey and his organization have many detractors, some claiming that he is too optimistic about how quickly solutions and repair technologies can be developed, but even more objecting that the aim of indefinite life extension is undesirable in itself. Zero Books is glad to have spoken to Aubrey de Grey, to have given him another opportunity to respond to critics and explain his project. This conversation took place over several weeks and was recorded in three sessions in October of 2015.

Douglas Lain, Zero Books

Part One

The Science of Indefinite Life Extension

Douglas Lain: I thought I'd start our conversation with a joke from Louis CK. Louis says that when you're forty and you go to the doctor, they don't try to fix anything anymore. Once you get over forty they don't try to fix you, they just say, "Yeah, that starts to happen." And they don't care. He says he went to doctor because his ankle hurt and the doctor showed him an x-ray and said: "Yeah, your ankle is just worn out. They get shitty like that when you're older. They're just not good anymore." I thought I'd start by asking if this is really a general attitude that people have, if doctors have that attitude, and if there is any truth in this joke.

Aubrey de Grey: Yes. There is an enormous amount of truth in it. And I think we need to distinguish here a little bit between the medical profession – doctors and other people in the medical world – as against the rest of the world. The medical profession have the enormous problem, which we need to sympathize with, that they have a certain range of tools to work with, to help people to be healthier and to restore people to health, but those tools are very limited in their efficacy. In particular they're extremely limited with regard to what they can do for people who are getting old. Ultimately, your average doctor just has to work with what they have, and a lot of that involves management of expectations. That's really all that Louis CK is saying there. Right?

Of course, that doesn't say anything about what might happen in the future. What might be possible in terms of maintenance or restoration of youthful good health with medicines that haven't yet been developed. But, that is not what doctors are supposed to be interested in. Doctors are all about doing their best with the tools that are already available.

Now contrast that with the situation that the general public has. The general public are not providing care, they are the recipient of medical care. And they are the people who should be thinking about the potential improvement in that medical care that might arise from further advances, from progress in the laboratory. It's kind of beholden on the public and therefore on policy makers and opinion formers and so on… to actually drive this, to actually deliver the funding and general resources that are required to allow people like SENS research foundation to move forward and create therapies that don't yet exist. Once those therapies do exist, of course they enter the universe of tools that your doctor can actually prescribe, can actually administer. But until that time, it's not the problem of the doctors. It's not their fault.

Douglas: So it's no surprise to you that doctors aren't turning to you now, you haven't developed anything that they… any tools for them to use yet.

Aubrey: You've got it. Doctors are using tools that already exist.

Douglas: Let's start then by defining our terms and figuring out the full scope of the project that your foundation SENS is working on. That's "Strategies for Engineering Negligible Senescence." That's what SENS stands for. What is aging? This is what you're fighting. What is aging and how do you and others who are working on achieving negligible senescence define that term and how does the scientific community think about aging, perhaps in contrast to how you think about it?

Aubrey: Aging is a really simple phenomenon. A lot of people in the broader world presume that aging is still a mystery, that nobody understands really what's going on. But that's bullshit. The actual fact is that people who study the biology of aging feel that they have a pretty good understanding of what's actually going on. Sure we could always get a better understanding, there are details that are still unclear, but at the end of the day the fundamentals are really well understood.

The aging of a human being, or any living organism, is actually really similar, really very similar, to the aging of an inanimate object like a car or an airplane. It's simply the accumulation of damage as a side effect of the machine's normal operation. So, in exactly the same way that a car will progressively accumulate rust and eventually the doors will fall off, similarly the human body accumulates... well, the equivalent of rust, various types of molecular and cellular damage, and eventually that damage accumulates to a level of abundance that is more than what the body is set up to tolerate. And that's when the overall function of the body starts to decline.

That's all that aging is. It's a really simple phenomenon. That's not controversial at all, you ask any gerontologist, any person who studies the biology of aging, what aging is, then they may use slightly different words, but essentially they'll say what I just said. Then the question is, what will we do about it? And certainly there are many different approaches that people have taken to that.

I believe the approach that SENS Research Foundation is taking, which is essentially a comprehensive damage-repair approach, is the most promising. But, some people have been working hard for a long time on the idea of simply slowing down the rate at which the body creates that damage in the first place. And that's another alternative. No question. It's another alternative. As things stand it looks to me very much as though that alternative is never going to work. It's not. It's far less practical than the damage-repair approach. But, we shall see.

Douglas: Maybe the people who are working on slowing down the damage that the body does to itself have a slightly different conception of what aging is. They tend to talk about changing the genes, almost like we have a clock that ticks through our lives, and then at a certain point the alarm goes off. Am I

misunderstanding this? Is there a slight difference here in the perspective on aging?

Aubrey: Yes you are misunderstanding. There is really no difference in perspective. Everyone understands that ultimately the reason why an older body works less well than a younger body is because the older body is carrying around more damage. The damage has come to exist as a result of the body's normal operation. The things that body has to do to keep us alive. There is really no controversy about that. The only real controversy is with regards to what is plausible in terms of dealing with that damage, in terms of making that damage go away, or slowing down the accumulation of that damage. So, the language that is often used, especially when gerontologists talk to the general public and journalists, may be a little misleading sometimes. Some of my colleagues, for example, let me pick out Cynthia Kenyon who is a good friend and an excellent scientist, but she sometimes is prone to use language that journalists misunderstand as in some way implying that aging is the consequence of some kind of program. She doesn't really mean that, she is just talking about the modulation, the ability of the body to modulate the rate of aging in response to certain pressures. And she'll often, of course, speak about her own work which is in very short-lived organisms. But, ultimately there is not a fundamental difference between her view and my view of what aging actually is.

Douglas: Have previous attempts to overcome aging... there's a long history of people working to defeat aging, going back to really pre-scientific times. Have previous attempts to overcome this process had a different conception of aging?

Aubrey: That's a great question. I really don't think they have. I think that even if you go back to Roger Bacon in the 1200s or whatever, you've still got an understanding that aging is a medical problem that should be amenable to medical intervention. And certainly if we go back to, for example, the '50s when the free-radical theory of aging was first put forward, that was the first really bona fide molecular theory of how aging actually goes on. And there, it was totally clear. Everyone understood, even back then, that the process of aging consists of the accumulation of damage.

Douglas: To me it seems like there are two different issues once you come to accept that aging is just this process where the body damages itself as it goes through its daily practices and that the damage is going to build up over time, and that when you start to think about intervening, the first thought that comes to mind is maybe not too realistic. It's about overcoming death. The other though is about extending our good health.

I can imagine that if there really was a program, there isn't, but if there was a program in the body somehow that just was set so that we all die at seventy-six years of age, that your kind of intervention, what you're talking about, would still be really worth investing in because even if you didn't extend life you would be improving people's health dramatically by undoing that damage.

Aubrey: Well you're right. Yeah.

There is an awful lot of talk around gerontologists about the idea of what they often call the compression of morbidity. In other words, essentially extending the healthy lifespan without similarly extending total lifespan. Therefore reducing the gap between the two, the amount of time that people spend at the end of life being unhealthy. That sounds terribly seductive and, of course, it's very politically correct and that's probably why so many of my colleagues have spent so much time highlighting their ideas that this might in principle be possible, but in practice it's not possible at all. Pretty much all of my colleagues accept perfectly well, that actually the only way we're ever going to extend lifespan is by extending healthspan, by extending healthy lifespan. That ultimately, being frail, being in a bad state of health, is always going to be risky. It's always going to be a state in which your likely future lifespan is short. Your likelihood of dying soon is high. Therefore, the only way we're ever going to get any kind of serious extension of lifespan is as a side effect of postponing ill health in the first place, in other words by extending healthy lifespan.

Douglas: And your organization is working on many things that will extend a healthy lifespan and that I would think people would be very excited about even if they're not truly interested in longevity. I saw a video presentation on your site about heart disease and macro-phages and undoing the damage done by oxidized cholesterol. I would think that you wouldn't have to be a gerontologist interested in longevity research but could just be a heart specialist and be very interested in what you're working on. So, how solid is the science behind that speculation and do you anticipate that this project might be able to contribute to breakthrough therapies before you get everything else in line to truly extend the lifespan?

Aubrey: You very cogently highlight the issue here – the relationship between the diseases of old age on the one hand and aging itself on the other hand. Essentially what you're really doing is highlighting the fact that there is no such thing as aging itself. In other words, that all of the aspects of the ill health of old age are intertwined. There is no real profit, no real merit, in trying to dissect them or to bifurcate that set of problems into things that are diseases on the one hand and things that are not diseases on the other hand. It's just... it's pointless. It makes no sense, and it's counterproductive because it makes people over-optimistic about some aspects of aging and unduly pessimistic about others.

In particular, if we look at, for example, the case that you mentioned of the role of oxidized cholesterol in driving heart disease then we can say, okay, yeah, heart disease is the number-one killer in the Western world and therefore if we could develop ways to enhance the robustness of white blood cells so they would be able to continue to process cholesterol without being poisoned by oxidized cholesterol the way they are today, then great! We might be able to more or less entirely prevent heart disease. But what would that mean in terms of the extension of healthy lifespan? Not a lot.

It turns out that, because of the exponential nature of the relationship between age and the risk of these diseases, we would only actually extend healthy lifespan by a few years, three or four years, before all the other things kicked in – cancer and Alzheimer's and so on – that were also increasing exponentially with age. We've got to hit the entire spectrum.

Douglas: I want to give you an opportunity to really lay out your perspective, especially this point about how you can't escape the diseases of old age without overcoming aging. That's very significant, but I'm so much on board with what you're doing that I'm looking for ways for you to get more support. It seems to me that there are people who might be reluctant to get involved in longevity research or working on all of these different pieces, but that if you could present this approach to the people who are working on heart disease, they would be very excited just in their little niche. I'm wondering if that is the case, or what the response to what you're doing is from those people.

Aubrey: Certainly it has been noticed that the real problem here is the relationship between how aging is perceived versus how the diseases of old age are perceived. We recognize that in order to majorly postpone the ill health of old age we would need to get all of these things working, reasonably effectively. That's a very tall order that isn't going to happen any time soon. So, for sure, it makes a lot sense to think about how we could appeal to the specific disease communities with regard to the effectiveness of these therapies against individual diseases. Let's just take heart disease as an example. Atherosclerosis is the ultimate driver of heart attacks and strokes, therefore it's the number-one killer in the Western world. We have this approach that involves bringing in new genes from bacteria that encode enzymes that will be able to break down oxidized cholesterol and therefore protect white blood cells in the artery wall from being poisoned by that contaminant. It's a great idea and it would certainly have an effect on atherosclerosis. We believe that it could be a much more potent therapy against atherosclerosis than anything that exists today.

But, there are a couple of issues there. The first issue is if we asked what the impact of that would be on longevity the answer is really small. The fact that all the diseases of old age have a progression that is exponentially related to age. In other words your chance of having Alzheimer's, for example, at age seventy-five is twice that at age seventy. And your chance of having it age eighty is twice what it was at age seventy-five. That is actually a real kicker when it comes longevity, because it means even if we completely eliminated atherosclerosis from the population it would still only extend people's healthy lifespan and therefore people's total lifespan by three or four years. That's a problem. The other problem is the way that… it's kind of related… the way that the disease community sees these things. If you have a therapy that postpones the ill health of atherosclerosis by five years, that is tantamount to a cure by most people's standards within the disease community, because they measure the effec-tiveness of their therapies under the assumption that no progress has been simultaneously made in postponing ill health from other diseases like cancer or Alzheimer's or whatever. This is a completely crazy assumption, but nevertheless it's the way they measure things. So, they don't think in terms of aiming as high as we're aiming.

Douglas: There are two hurdles to overcome in the thinking that's going on right now in the medical community or in the scientific community. The first one is just... there is a lot of resistance, for a variety of reasons, to longevity as a goal or to tackling the damage that the body does to itself or just to do something about aging or intervening in that process directly. There is a lot of resistance to that. But then, there is also seemingly a resistance to just this damage-repair model itself. To what extent is this approach, this maintenance model, in play in the medical community now? How much of this type of thinking is going on just when it comes to treating diseases rather than something big and systemic like aging?

Aubrey: Great question. Both within the medical disease-specific community and within the gerontology community the idea of damage repair is kind of a Cinderella concept. Because on the one hand people understand that in the ideal world it would be the Holy Grail, it would be the way to go. You would be able to take people who are already suffering from this or that condition, or are close to suffering from it, and you would be able to turn the clock backwards and get to the point where they were, essentially, in a youthful condition whether in relation to a specific disease or in relation to all aspects of age-related ill health, but the issue is how you do it. And the only reason I was able to come along fifteen years ago and put this idea forward is because I brought together a whole bunch of ideas that came from a wide variety of different areas of biology.

Biology, and this is true of the whole of science but perhaps it's worse in biology than it is elsewhere, is ridiculously Balkanized.

In other words, your typical biologist knows about their own stuff and about stuff that is closely related to their own work, but knows nothing to speak of about what is going on in other areas of biology. It's just the nature of how science works especially in the modern era where science is so poorly funded and therefore people have so little opportunity to spend their time exploring areas at the periphery of their preexisting expertise.

I was able to escape that phenomenon. I was able to explore broadly, because I was able to create my own career essentially in my spare time, but it's extraordinarily rare for that to be the case. We have this really bad situation of bias of the whole system against cross-disciplinary work, and SENS is about as cross-disciplinary as it comes. I mean, the whole idea of bringing additional genes into the whole area of treating atherosclerosis, that idea comes from something that wasn't originally bio-medical at all. It was actually from environmental decontamination, from an area called Bioremediation. You know, something completely different.

Douglas: Why is it that a cross-disciplinary approach is so vitally important to a maintenance approach?

Aubrey: That's easy to say. It's simply that the damage repair is inherently cross-disciplinary because the damage itself is inherently heterogeneous. The body does so much... so many different types of damage to itself at the molecular and cellular level and we've got to settle them all in order to get significant increase in the postponement of ill health in old age.

Douglas: Right, but do we have to tackle them all in order to overcome heart disease?

Aubrey: Oh, yes we do. I mean basically all these are wrapped up in each other. So you could say well no, we only have to do one of them in order to deal with heart disease, but so what really? Even if we don't have any heart disease at all we would still only extend longevity by a few years because we get these other diseases. You know, increasing exponentially with age, same as heart disease.

Douglas: I guess I think that getting the money from the disease people would be a good idea and if you could do the maintenance on just on heart disease that you'd get a whole lot of support on that. But getting to the point to get people to even think about maintenance is difficult for the reasons you mentioned.

Aubrey: That's right. And let me explain another difficulty. The disease community – because they only look at their own disease and they measure success in terms of the postponement of their own disease, on the assumption that other diseases are not postponed – the problem is that they are overly interested in really minor progress. Even in small amounts of progress. We aren't.

We're interested in major progress, and of course, it's harder to make big progress than it is to make small progress. So if you go to people who are focused on a particular disease they're not going to be very interested in what we're doing. They're saying, "Oh, that's too hard. Let's do easier stuff," because they're going to be focused on the modest benefit of the easier stuff and they're not going to think of that as unacceptably modest.

Douglas: Right. And this was something that I heard in... I'm not sure which debate it was. I watched you debate a bunch of different people. There was a gerontologist who was fairly angry with you because he thought your optimism and your ambition was going to possibly mean that dollars that could to be sent to him and his people to do this sort of minor research

that was realistic and necessary would be diverted to your pie-in-the-sky organization. **What would you say to those people who are trying to be more modest? And to him?**

Aubrey: The same thing, really. It's like... these people are politically correct. They're politically reluctant to even talk about the idea of major progress because they feel that policy makers and opinion formers will be unimpressed. They feel that those people will just say, "Well, this is obviously science fiction." So, in other words it will bring the whole field into disrepute. Of course that's a very short-sighted way of thinking about it. If my colleagues were willing to actually look at the logic and understand that it doesn't mean that at all, but actually the prospect of extending the human lifespan is actually extremely realistic, then people would say, "Well okay, everyone is saying it's realistic therefore it probably is realistic, therefore we shouldn't think of it as science fiction." But unfortunately they aren't thinking of it in that way.

Douglas: So you think it's very realistic. There are a lot of people who are resistant to that. I'll give you the opportunity now to kind of go over your approach and what the problems are, the seven different problems that need to be overcome, and why you think it is a realistic approach to coping with the diseases related to old age and to aging itself. What are those approaches and why are they realistic?

Aubrey: The answer to that comes in two parts. On the one hand we have to ask: Is it realistic that we could develop the technologies that SENS Research Foundation currently talks about and pursues? The technologies of SENS, and that's all about the first steps of getting rid of damage. So, I've always said that I think these technologies will give us only a few decades of additional healthy life, perhaps thirty years of healthy life.

Which is an awful lot compared to what anyone's achieved so far regarding the diseases and disability of old age, but still it is actually, you know, relatively unscary from a demographic point of view and in terms of the other things people tend to come up with.

The reason why people tend to get so intimidated by what I talk about is because I look one step further. I say: Well hang on, since these therapies are bona-fide rejuvenation therapies that we're proposing to invent, since they'll be applied to people who are already in middle age or older when they're developed, and they will give those people an additional thirty years of healthy life, we have to take into account what's going to happen next... what's going to happen over the subsequent thirty years? Those thirty years before those people get back to being biologically sixty. And thirty years is one hell of a long time in terms of technology, in terms of any technology and certainly in terms of medical technology. So the question is, what do we do about that? I feel, very clearly, that the thirty years that we have there will be easily enough for us to improve the comprehensiveness and performance of those therapies such that we will be able to take the same people, the people who got the first generation therapies, and re-rejuvenate them at age ninety when they're biologically sixty for the second time, right? So they will not be biologically sixty for the third time until they are chronologically, let's say, a hundred and fifty. And so on.

This is the thing that I've called longevity escape velocity. And that's what leads me to the conclusion that it's highly likely that a lot of people who are alive today will actually live way beyond a hundred and twenty, or a hundred and fifty, in fact into four-digit lifespans if not longer. This is something that really frightens the horses. It's something that the more politically correct members of my community have really recoiled from, despite the ineluctable logic of it, because they feel it's going to go down very poorly in the corridors of power.

I think that is a ridiculously short-sighted and cowardly approach and attitude, but there it is.

Douglas: Why is it politically correct to avoid that? I guess because you don't want it to sound like science fiction when you're proposing a realm of research, but beyond that if you do start to see that your logic is correct and that this is feasible, what is it that makes it politically correct?

Aubrey: It's very simple. Most politicians, in fact almost all politicians, have one objective in mind. Namely, getting re-elected. They don't lead public opinion, they follow public opinion. The question is, what is public opinion? Of course, public opinion consists of the opinions of people who are not terribly capable of following an argument as subtle as the one I just gave you. These are people who will look at the conclusion of the argument, namely the thousand-year lifespan or whatever, and they'll say "Oh, dear this is complete science fiction let's ignore it." Without actually taking the trouble to see how that conclusion was arrived at. And, you know, it's perfectly reasonable. If, ultimately, you are interested in getting funding, public funding, it's perfectly reasonable to pander to that. It's reasonable to feel that, maybe it's true, maybe it's not true, people in general are going to feel that it's not true, and therefore if you support it you're going to damage your own chances at public funding. I'm sympathetic to that. I understand that most of my colleagues are ultimately not able to be real scientists anymore. They are ultimately doing what they do as a career, and I'm extremely privileged to be able to tell the truth.

Douglas: Let me ask you a question about the feasibility of your approach. Let's say that there weren't any advances in this maintenance approach. You developed a maintenance approach that gave you thirty years and that's as far as it went.

Would you be able to, in thirty years, implement the same intervention and have a similar result, where you get another thirty years? Is there a reason why you can't keep doubling down on the same treatment? Would it just mean that it would just slow down the aging process so that you would get fifteen years the next time?

Aubrey: I'm trying to understand your question. It sounds like it's circular. It sounds like "If this couldn't be done could it be done?"

Douglas: You've created an approach that gives us thirty years more. That's done. For escape velocity you say that there will be a lot more improvements. I'm suggesting that over those years there wouldn't be improvements, but there would still be the original intervention.

Aubrey: What you are overlooking, or rather what I didn't say yet, is the frequency with which one actually administers the first-generation therapy. I didn't say that those therapies are administered once and then in thirty years the person is back at biologically the same age as they were thirty years previously. The frequency of the administration of the therapies may be quite high. It may be every year, it may be every day even, depending on how they're administered. We just don't know the details of that. The reason why the therapies would only deliver a certain finite amount of extension of healthy lifespan is because of the gaps that they have. So, in other words what you would have is, people would have a level of health that is determined by the total level of damage of these various categories, but within each category there are subcategories and some are easy to fix and some subcategories are difficult to fix. So, let us, for the sake of argument, simply partition the subcategories according to whether they are fixed by the first-generation therapies. Right? What we have is, you've got your person. Let's say they're sixty.

They get the first-generation therapies and those first-generation therapies work on some of the various subcategories of damage in each category and not on the others. And then, the reason those people get back to being biologically sixty at the age of being chronologically ninety is because they have accumulated an amount of damage that falls into the subcategories that the therapies don't work on that is equal to what the person had in total at age sixty without the therapy. So they've got essentially zero amount of easy damage, but they've got maybe twice as much difficult damage as what they had at age sixty and that leads them to a level of total damage that is equal to what they had at age sixty before the therapies came along.

Douglas: Hearing you say that it seems like the consequences of that new more difficult damage are not going to be exactly the same—

Aubrey: No. That's not true. The consequences are going to be pretty much the same. Let me give you a concrete example of this. Let's take hypertension. Hypertension is something that increases with age, and the main reason it increases with age is because of what's called glycation. The process of accumulation of chemical bonds between the proteins in the lattice of structures called the extracellular matrix. The extracellular matrix is the lattice of proteins that gives our tissues their elasticity, and elasticity is really important in the skin to stop wrinkles; it's important in the lens of the eye so that we can see close-up because of the need to deform the shape of the lens; and most life-threateningly it's important in the major arteries in order to dampen the oscillation of blood pressure that comes from the heartbeat and protect the more fragile components of the circulation capillaries. So it's really important for that elasticity to be maintained, and it is not maintained. We accumulate crosslinking. Now the reason I'm mentioning this one, there are different structures that accumulate, a bunch of different types of chemical structures that bind together and reduce elasticity. At this point, we at SENS Research Foundation are going after the number-one contributor, the one that constitutes the largest proportion of those crosslinks. It's called glucosepane and we are doing very well. In fact, just yesterday we had a paper in *Science* magazine that is a really great step towards getting rid of this stuff.

But, the point is, when we do get rid of it, there is still a bunch of other structures that are also accumulating, and eventually on their own, even in the absence of this number-one structure, their total contribution to stiffness of the artery wall will be enough to be problematic. The point is, however, we have plenty of time before that happens. But, the overall consequence of that stiffening is exactly the same as what we see today before we get rid of the number-one problem.

So it's all a matter of simply controlling the pathologies by controlling the damage that leads to the pathologies one step at a time.

Douglas: I want to dig in a little bit on this question of feasibility from a different direction, one that I'm more comfortable with since I'm not a scientist. Which is just, what do people in authority say about your research. Ten years ago there was a contest wherein $20,000 was offered to any molecular biologist who could prove that the alleged benefits of SENS were so wrong that they were not worthy of learned debate.

Aubrey: That's right. In fact, we put up half of that money.

Douglas: And there were three competitors but none of them collected the $20,000. Could you summarize what kinds of arguments were given and why they failed to persuasively argue against debating or researching SENS?

Aubrey: Sure. Yeah. We actually provided half of the prize fund because we knew that it was vital to smoke out the opposition. Prior to that time there had been an abundance of off-the-record ridicule which indeed had led to the magazine that you're talking about, *MIT Technology Review*, coming to a completely unwarranted conclusion with regard to the implausibility of SENS. And that's why they were interested in coming to a more justified conclusion.

So, of the three entries that came in, two of them were basically just complete wastes of time. They were just based on complete misunderstandings of what SENS actually said. And so they kind of... they were irrelevant.

But the third entry, which was an entry authored by nine people, most of whom were very credentialed gerontologists. That was much more interesting. The reason it was interesting was because it did start from a basic understanding of what we were trying to say on the nature of damage repair. The objections that were given in that challenge were all about whether specific components of the damage-repair approach could actually realistically be implemented in the foreseeable future. And the reason why that challenge was thrown out, very unceremoniously by the neutral experts who were appointed to adjudicate, was very straightforward. It was just that the authors didn't know enough. That they had not taken the trouble to read my papers, in particular to read the references, the experimental work that I'd cited in my papers. And therefore they were unaware of how close we already were to implementing these things, and therefore how realistic it was to get from where we already were to where we needed to be.

Douglas: So, this was the Estep... he was the main author. One argument that I could understand when I looked through what he said was that he said you ignored important scientific studies that might cast doubt on your hypothesis and the feasi-

bility of your ideas. He said you were cherry picking. And then you responded that this was not the case and he responded that it was. Do you care to talk about that accusation at all?

Aubrey: Well… of course I was right and he was wrong.

Douglas: It doesn't help very much to hear you say that.

Aubrey: Otherwise the judges would not have come to the conclusion that they came to.

Douglas: Okay. Okay. But did he get some money in the end? Did they give him half of the prize or something?

Aubrey: That was rather interesting. The editor of the *Technology Review*, Jason Pontin… he had come to an intuitive conclusion that I must be talking complete bullshit and he had really laid himself on the line by writing a couple of extremely derogatory and rude editorials in the, I think, February 2005 issue of the magazine, accompanying a profile on me. So, he basically nailed his colors very much to the mast. And the result is that after what happened he had a fabulously enormous face-saving exercise to engage in. Which he is still engaged in to be honest. He hasn't actually, even ten years later, really come to terms with the fact that he got it wrong back then.

Douglas: The strange thing is that Preston Estep is not a critic of the idea of life extension itself, as far as I can tell from trying to research him a little bit. According to the notoriously unreliable Wikipedia, what I found out is that he advocates mind uploading as an approach to overcoming aging and death.
Is that true? Do you know what his overall stance is toward aging?

Aubrey: I don't know what he thinks of mind uploading, but I do understand that he is in favor of defeating aging in general as a goal. It's just that he doesn't feel that our approach is feasible. And his rationale for dismissing our approach is not terribly well justified.

Douglas: Well that's interesting to me because most of the time when your critics... your critics usually say two things at once. Critics say that it's completely infeasible and it's not desirable. But, he didn't say that. That doesn't mean it's right. What was his main criticism?

Aubrey: I could spend a half an hour being rude about Estep. The fact is he just didn't read enough.

But you're absolutely right, a lot of people are much more messed up in terms of their reaction to all this than Estep was. Because as you say, they say both these things. They say this is infeasible and it's undesirable. And they don't realize what they're doing. They don't realize that actually they are resisting the imperative to actually decide whether it is feasible, because they've decided that it doesn't matter whether it's feasible because it's a bad idea. And at the same time they are resisting the ideas that it might be a good idea because they've decided it's infeasible.

So I spend an awful lot of my time, when debating these people like Colin Blakemore for example, trying to embarrass them into realizing no, you can't do this, it's intellectually bankrupt. It's embarrassing to combine these things. You've got to address these two questions – the desirability and the feasibility – separately from each other.

Douglas: I want to give you the opportunity to really give your more... what to me anyway was one of your more convincing arguments, which was when you just go through the seven

21

types of damage that we need to repair in order to lengthen our lifespan.

Aubrey: I think you're asking the wrong question there. We do have this seven-point plan that SENS Research Foundation is pursuing, but really I think the important thing is not so much to enumerate what the seven components are, the important thing is to deal with a justification for why it's a good plan. And there are two components to that. One part is whether it's a sufficient plan. In other words, whether there might be some kind of eighth category that we haven't identified that will kill us on schedule even if we fix all the existing seven. And the other question is whether it's a necessary plan, whether there is some way to sidestep all of this and postpone the ill health of old age in some much simpler way. And I believe that both of those questions are really important. We are indeed addressing them in projects that we are funding. With regard to whether the plan is sufficient, there is plenty of circumstantial evidence. We can just look at the fact that, historically within the field, within the studies of the biology of aging, all seven of the things we point to are problems that have been major topics within gerontology for more than thirty years. That's a very long time. You kind of think that if there was a number eight coming along it should have come by now. It's been twelve years at least since I've been going out there making a nuisance of myself and challenging people to actually come up with a category number eight. And that hasn't elicited an example either. I seem to be getting away with it. Again, it's looking pretty good. Now of course, you could say, "Well, hang on. That's only circumstantial evidence." And I agree it is only circumstantial, but hey, you know, what do you need? We could argue that the only way to identify category number eight is to fix the other seven and then see what happens in mice. See if they die on schedule. If they do then we'll be able to see why. We'll be able to unmask category number eight. That's a perfectly good research strategy. Then when we come to the other question of whether there might be a simpler way to go... I mean this is a really important thing, because of course the whole of gerontology, and the position of gerontology before I came along, was focused on exactly that. It was focused, and still is focused overwhelmingly, on the idea that we might be able to identify some kind of magic bullet. We've seen in various short-lived organisms really simple ways to extend longevity by a lot, by just changing one gene or by starvation or whatever, and that's interesting. The only reason that we feel that that is not the way to go for the human body is because it doesn't seem to scale. There are very good reasons, both theoretical and now experimental, to believe that longer-lived organisms will benefit far less from these magic bullets than mice or worms or whatever actually do. So it's a source of great frustration to me that the field, including the private sector – just for example Calico, the company that Google set up – are apparently still fixated on the idea that there might be these simple approaches that might work.

Douglas: I think that it might go back to what we were talking about at the very beginning of this conversation, this desire to find a simple clock that we can set back. Maybe the genes would be that clock.

I don't know. That may be far afield of what they're thinking.

Aubrey: Well, no. That's pretty much what they are thinking. That's right. I'm not a fan of wishful thinking. I'm more interested in actually getting results.

Part Two

Pick One – Infeasible or Inadvisable?

Douglas: I thought we'd talk today about the desirability of life extension and the SENS project. We'll begin with this: What I've noticed is that in the debates that you've had on this subject, the ones I can find on YouTube, your opponents have a peculiar knack for undermining their own position. When I was a kid I used to argue with my religious friends in Colorado Springs, and I'd try to convince them there was no God. I'd say things like, "Look, God doesn't exist and besides, he's an idiot." You get the same approach. People will say that not only is the idea of intervening to repair the damage done to the body by aging a pipe dream or impossible, it's also just inadvisable. It's a bad idea.

Aubrey: That's right. That's certainly what they say.

Douglas: What do you think accounts for this approach? It's common to scientists and lay people alike. Why are they doing this? Why is this so common?

Aubrey: Well I think the problem is that the two issues exacerbate and reinforce each other. In other words, people have basically been brought up to be dismissive of both the desirability and the feasibility of doing anything about aging. And therefore they will kind of refuse to think about either of them because they're already convinced about the other one. You know, they will not really pay much attention to discussions of whether the defeat of aging is a good idea because they'll say, "Well who cares if it's a good idea, it's obviously impossible and therefore it's just an academic question." But at the same time the same people will be very reluctant to pay much attention to conversations about whether the whole thing is possible because they've already decided that it's a bad idea. They'll say, "Well, so what if it's possible? We wouldn't want to do it anyway." So, I spend an awful lot of my time essentially embarrassing people into assessing these questions separately from each other and thereby giving themselves the opportunity to actually make some progress.

Douglas: Do you think that people are holding onto an idea about there being such a thing as a natural death because of their fear of getting old and getting very ill, or is there some other reason why people would want to hold onto aging and death as some sort of natural limit that we shouldn't try to pass.

Aubrey: I think probably the number-one thing that drives all of this is fear of getting their hopes up. Having made their peace with the idea that there is this inevitable albeit ghastly thing that's going to happen to them in the distant future, they want simply to put it out of their minds and not reengage that question and be preoccupied by it. Because they know that if they form the opinion that there is some chance that they will escape this fate, that nobody has escaped so far, then they might end up being wrong because progress in the relevant medical research might not be quite as fast as that. They just prefer to carry on believing, or pretending, that the whole thing is completely impossible and any discussion to the contrary is fanciful, because it allows to get on with their miserably short lives and make the best of it.

Douglas: Right... are you aware of this writer Ernest Becker? Have you ever heard of him?

Aubrey: No.

Douglas: He wrote a book in the '70s called *The Denial of Death*.

Aubrey: All right. I recognize the name of the book, but I haven't read it.

Douglas: The premise there is that not only is the denial of death important to understand for a psychologist, but in fact this denial of death explains human behavior on the cultural level. It's really what's driving us to create culture itself.

I wonder if you think it's possible that there is more riding on a belief in the naturalness of death than merely a way to put the misery of life out of one's head? Do we sort of rely on this natural limit in some other way?

Aubrey: Yeah, I don't know. I'm definitely not a psychologist. I'm just basing my opinions on what people say when I talk to them about this.

I mean, as you say, it's just absurd how illogical people will be, including the educated people who make their living out of being logical. It's bewildering.

Douglas: Do you find that to be the case especially among people who are actually working on aging, like gerontologists?

Aubrey: Oh, not at all. No. Almost all gerontologists are perfectly sane about this. They understand that aging is bad for you and that we ought to do something about it.

For quite a while during the 1970s and '80s especially, and really through the '90s, it was kind of a view that dare not speak its name. It was something that was very much swept under the carpet. In grant applications or interviews and so on, senior gerontologist would almost all shy away from all this, and talk about aging as a phenomenon to be studied in order to understand it better without any particular emphasis on doing anything about it. But, very thankfully, that is more or less over. Now it is absolutely normal, however credentialed and mainstream, to discuss the postponement of age-related ill health as a very real and very legitimate goal.

The disputes that happen within gerontology revolve pretty much entirely around the question of which is the most promising approach to doing that.

Douglas: Is that because the science caught up? Now they can be more optimistic and not be thought of as engaging in fantasy?

Aubrey: I'm not really sure that it's because the science caught up. I would like to think my own advocacy played a certain role. I've had a high profile throughout all of this time. I have made a lot of noise about how embarrassingly illogical it is to deny that aging is bad for you, and perhaps that has progressively rubbed off and it's become more embarrassing to take the historical position that aging is just this thing to be understood than it is to take the contrary position that aging is something to be manipulated.

Douglas: The people who do argue that we shouldn't desire to extend the human lifespan indefinitely, what are their major objections? Is the first one that you hear involving population and overpopulation as a concern?

Aubrey: That is the most common, yes. People have this fabulously immediate knee-jerk reaction that "Oh, God. If we eliminated aging then instantly we'd have a population problem that would be absolutely unmanageable." So much so that we actually ended up funding an entire study done by a very credentialed group at the University of Denver, who have a system that's been developed for over thirty years that's used by the United Nations and many other authoritative governmental and non-governmental groups. We paid them to extend the versatility of their system so that they could look at a world in which aging was under complete medical control. And the main purpose was of course to dispel all this, to actually put proper numbers behind what was likely to be the actual trajectory of global population, and thereby, of course, to show that the rise in population, which will happen, will be slow enough that it's very unlikely indeed that we will be outrun by the improvement that technology gives us in terms of the carrying capacity of the planet, by reducing pollution and so on. This will happen because of the move toward renewable energy, for example.

Douglas: I think there is a lot of pessimism about the possibilities for renewable energy. Even if you take the possibility of indefinite lifespan off the table, I think there are many people today who feel that we're headed for a population crisis and we're just going to use up the planet. Doom and gloom is pretty pervasive, especially on the left side of the spectrum. What would you say to people who had those concerns?

Aubrey: Well, it's kind of the same concern. The question is will this actually happen? One can always point to other things like the fertility rates come down as time goes on, because as any particular society gets wealthier and women have more education and emancipation and so on, that they just choose to have fewer children and choose to have children later. I believe actually that technology-based increase in the carrying capacity of the Earth is the biggest factor, the fact that is going to make the greatest difference and obviate and let us avoid any serious problems of overpopulation, even the problems that we have today before there has been any progress against aging.

Douglas: I think if your techniques [against aging] work that would be a pretty strong argument for the power of technology to overcome problems. Now the other kinds of objections that

you get are, I think, so specious that they're really not worth talking about too much. There is the objection that people will never leave seats of power, or that younger people will never find a good position in society, but those objections are incredibly weak because the benefits of life extension far outweigh those problems even if they continue. Do you want to address any big objections that come up that I didn't mention?

Aubrey: I mean, of course I could go through a million different objections and talk about them individually. One particularly laughable one is that we might have dictators living forever, which is particularly hilarious because dictator tends to rank pretty high on the league table of risky jobs. The people who get those jobs don't typically die of aging. And when they do die from aging that doesn't work because they tend to be able to orchestrate their succession as well. The individual arguments, rebutting these concerns, are all very well. I think it makes sense to actually do that, but not necessarily for people like me to do it. I think what really matters is for people who are the experts in the various areas to do it. You know? Whether it's economics or sociology or agriculture or whatever.

What I would, however, like to add are two arguments that are kind of universal. They kind of transcend all of the specific concerns that people come up with.

The first one is "sense of proportion."

People are very inclined to come up with this or that potential problem that might be created as a consequence of solving the problem we have today, the problem of age-related ill health, and they'll immediately switch their brains off and say let's not do it. But, of course, the question is: Even in the worst-case scenario where this problem did occur and we were unable to address it by some specific approach, would the problem be worse than the problem we have today? And in order to answer that question one has to actually quantify, in one's own mind, how bad the problem is that we have today. I feel that's rather easy, just look at the number of deaths and furthermore the fact that it's 100,000 people a day and furthermore that most of those people are dying after a period, a long period, of general decline and disease, and decrepitude, and dependence, and general misery. Right? That to me is a pretty uninspired argument. We should not be allowing ourselves to hesitate on the basis of uncertainty about what would result.

The second argument, which is perhaps even more ironclad, is with regard to who has the entitlement to make the choice. Because basically what we're saying here is that we, humanity of today, have the option either to develop these therapies as fast as we can or not to. And if we don't, if we say "Oh dear, overpopulation, dictators living forever, let's not go there," and we hesitate and prevaricate, then that will, of course, delay (not indefinitely by any means, but it will delay) the arrival of these therapies. And that, of course, means that a certain sector, a certain cohort of humanity, will be condemned to the same kind of painful and early death that humanity has suffered historically, when, in practice, they could have benefited from escaping all that on account of the therapies having been developed in time for them. So the question is:

Do we have the right to make that choice? It seems perfectly clear to me that we don't. The people who are entitled to make that choice are the people of the future who will, apart from anything else, have better information with regard to which technologies, whether it's renewable energy, nuclear fusion, artificial meat, or whatever... which of those technologies have actually been developed and therefore which of the potential, hypothetical problems, that might be created or prevented by curing aging, has actually been averted. They can choose whether to actually use these therapies, and if so how to use them, on the basis of the information available to them, rather than be condemned to live with the choices that their ancestors made.

Douglas: Both of those are strong arguments against the basic objections that you get.

I wanted to bring up one more objection that I found, and it was in the journal called "EMBO Reports." It was a paper written about a decade ago by Charles McConnel and Lee Turner, and it was entitled "Medicine, Aging, and Longevity." They mentioned you in the article. It seems to me that they misrepresent your aims a bit, and I'll give you a chance to address that. They say that your concept of engineered negligible senescence is linked to a vision in which all biological processes are "halted or reversed," but you're not really aiming at halting the aging process.

Aubrey: It's a little bit semantic. I mean, yes the particular approaches that we are developing constitute reversal of aging in the sense of repairing the damage that constitutes aging, and thereby restoring the molecular and cellular structure and composition of the body to something like what it was in an earlier age. The idea is to do that periodically so as to essentially counteract the ongoing creation of damage that the body is doing to itself in the process of its normal operation.

You know, whether one calls that reversing aging or halting aging it doesn't really matter, it's just semantic.

Douglas: So, here is what I think is the relevant quote from the paper:

"Epidemiologists and public health scholars challenge the widespread faith that gene therapy, stem-cell research and regenerative medicine will one day lead to substantial gains in human longevity. They argue that humans are complex biological organisms situated within particular economic, political, social and cultural environments and that ageing is a multifactorial, multidimensional process

unlikely to be significantly influenced at the population level by gene transfer or other biomedical technologies. By contrast, some bio-demographers note that due to the potentially devastating consequences of emerging lethal viruses, nutritional excesses, and deteriorating social and economic environments, average life expectancy may very well decline in the future."

So this is not really an objection to intervening, but just suggesting that it's not likely to be successful, but for strange reasons. I wanted to give you a chance to respond to it.

Aubrey: Yeah. Well, of course, I have absolutely no time for that kind of attitude. The idea is, "Oh dear, this is a hard problem. Let's all just wring our hands and not bother to try." That's not really my style.

Douglas: What do you make of the fact that they talk about "biological organisms situated within particular economic, political, social and cultural environments?"

Aubrey: They have a point. It makes the problem that much harder, we've got to figure out how to get these things available to people. Some people argue that, for example, the FDA is a barrier to that because it doesn't regard aging as a disease. I think that argument is overblown.

But, those kinds of things, those kinds of inherent aspects of inertia certainly exist. Of course, the biggest one of all is the inertia that exists because of what we were talking about earlier, the fear of getting one's hopes up, because that is something that leads to a lot of reluctance to actually put serious effort into the crusade against aging. Of course, SENS Research Foundation is at the sharp end of that reluctance because we don't have nearly as much money as we need to get the research done. The research is going much more slowly than it could as a result.

Douglas: The quote seemed to me to be pessimistic not only about the possibility for an indefinite life extension, but also about solving social problems in general.
There are "lethal viruses, nutritional excesses" and deficiencies really… and all these things, you know, for instance the "deteriorating social and economic environments," it's all just taken for granted that these things can't be overcome.

Aubrey: I think the only real way to look at this is to look at historical precedent. The obvious one to take, of course, is the Industrial Revolution. It was quite a shock to the system, it was quite turbulent, but there are very few people who would regard it in the long run as having been a bad idea. Most think it was quite a good idea. That's because we figured out how to muddle through and solve these various issues that come up as a result of the changes to society that were motivated by the introduction of these new technologies. As far as I'm concerned it's going to be exactly the same as that.

Douglas: Now in a presentation you gave at Transvision in 2014 you said that questions about human nature and the kinds of social and political changes that these achievements might bring should not be the major thing that people talked about, because it was quite easy to argue just based on sort of the normal understanding of the world and what a human being is that this is a good idea.
But, I'm just wondering if in this context, because this is going to be for a left press, if you might be willing to take a stab at discussing the changes that you think might be necessitated by an indefinite life extension, and then also just what your vision is for a world in which this has taken place. What do you see the future possibly being like?

Aubrey: It's difficult for me to answer that question directly. The first thing that I have difficulty with is the idea of thinking of anything really being necessitated. I think in terms of the amount of technology, and the creation of new technologies, as being something that increases the choice that humanity has. In other words things becoming available rather than not being available. So necessitating is kind of the opposite of what's going to happen.

But also, yes I have some kind of vague intuition about how things are going to be, but I know very well that such intuition has very little basis in fact. You know, ultimately I have no idea what the world is going to be like in twenty years let alone fifty years, because there are a whole bunch of other things that are going to happen in terms of, for example, the advance in automation, that are going to change the world really, really, radically even before the therapies that SENS Research Foundation are working on come to fruition.

I kind of feel that one needs to take a step back from this idea of envisioning how the world will be. One simply wants to look at properties of how the world will be that might be desirable or undesirable and the only property that really matters here is people won't get sick as a result of having been born a long time ago. There simply won't be any Alzheimer's disease. There will be hardly any cancer. There will be no osteoporosis or arteriosclerosis or whatever. And this sounds like a fairly unequivocal good thing. There are not many people who are in favor of the diseases of old age. So the main difficulty we have in persuading people that the whole endeavor is a good idea arises from just one thing, namely the bizarre Chinese wall that exists in people's minds as the difference between what they think of as aging itself as opposed to what they think of as the diseases of old age. There is absolutely zero biological, biomedical basis for that dichotomy. It's a false dichotomy, and when people understand it's a false dichotomy the whole question of whether this would be a good idea basically goes away in one go.

Douglas: I bring this up because working on the left, in left publishing, I've noticed that there is a resistance these days to envisioning a future and thinking seriously about structural change. What we get instead often are complaints about inequities that are happening now, which are justified often, but without any ambition to get at the roots of problems and no optimism about the likelihood of real systemic change.

It seems to me that your proposal here with SENS, if that were to happen, it does seem to me that it would necessitate some changes. I don't know exactly what they would be, but one that comes to mind is that people who are working in fields or in jobs that they don't enjoy and that are rather miserable, would be less likely to put up with that if they had the prospect of living a whole lot longer in those positions.

Bringing up automation there is another pressure to change the way people work, so I'm wondering if you think that that kind of positive change might be a byproduct of what you're doing medically.

Aubrey: Let's speculate about this.

Of course, I'm very much in favor of greater equality, of helping the disadvantaged to do better. If we look at the Gates Foundation, the biggest philanthropic organization in the world, they very much set their store, what they do is they help the disadvantaged. And it would be very difficult for SENS Research Foundation to get money out of the Gates Foundation because we're focusing on improving the lives of the leading edge rather than the trailing edge. And that's fine. I definitely want more mosquito nets in sub-Saharan Africa and so on.

It's kind of a category error, if you like, to try to call this an either/or. To try to say, "Oh we should try to help the disadvantaged before we start thinking about the technologies that might let people live a lot longer, or stop people from getting Alzheimer's however long they live." You know, that's just crazy because it's completely different expertise that's involved. It's completely different people who are involved in actually pursuing these objectives. It's not even the same money because different people are interested in different things and therefore different people will give money to these things. You know we've got money funding SENS Research Foundation that comes from people who have never given money to any kind of bio-medical charity of any kind before, just because we were the ones who actually inspired them.

I just don't think that it makes sense to regard this as any kind of dichotomy, or any kind of choice. It's a matter of let's do both things and get on with them.

Douglas: Right. I don't think it's a simple choice either, and I'd be the last person to suggest that we shouldn't focus on helping the disadvantaged. Obviously, that's necessary. And I do think your research should be supported as well. But, I also think that if the kinds of changes that your research represents were implemented that what it would mean to be disadvantaged may radically change for the better.

There was a presidential candidate who once said, I think it was George Bush who said, "We need to make the pie higher."

Just as the Industrial Revolution really changed the game and changed our expectations about what we could do, and what kind of lives we could have, research like yours might have the same consequence.

Aubrey: I agree, but I don't have deep thoughts about it.

Douglas: You're associated with transhumanism...

Aubrey: I'm not...

Douglas: ...in people's minds. I know that you're not officially

associated with them. But do you share some of those goals just personally, like the development of artificial intelligence? I know you used to work on that. Are you excited by the prospect of space travel?

Aubrey: I'm definitely a techno-visionary. I definitely believe that there are many areas of technology, of pioneering technology, that have the potential in the next few decades to transform humanity and the quality of human life... the human condition. Certainly the one that I'm working on, the elimination of aging, is by no means the only one.

Now, in that sense you could say that I am a transhumanist because I would say that if one actually comes up with a definition of what makes transhumanists like each other and hang out with each other, it is that. It's that they're in favor of pioneering radical new technologies. What I take issue with in regards to transhumanism is simply the "ism" aspect. It seems to me the best way to think about these radical, pioneering technologies, and indeed to talk about them, is to emphasize the continuity. The fact that these are things that are natural progressions from what we've done in the past in terms of technology. And that's not the way that transhumanism tends to be sold. Transhumanism tends to be sold as some kind of radical departure from normal thinking, which it really shouldn't be.

Douglas: So, I'm going to go back to the psychological barriers that may exist, and given how this conversation has gone so far I'm not sure how many comments you're going to have on some of these questions I'm going to ask you here, but we'll see.

It just strikes me that in general when humanity has had successes and gained mastery over the world, that's always come along with a kind of series of deflationary experiences. A long time ago we thought we were at the center of the universe but as we learned more we found out that we're on a tiny speck in a tiny speck. You know? We're nowhere close to being the center of anything. We thought we were God's creation but then we find out that we're just animals that evolved out of slime. Do you think that one of the reasons why you face opposition is because there is a deflationary impact on people as we gain mastery over the body, and that they're having to give up a sense of nature which might be supporting them?

Aubrey: I'm not sure I understand what you mean by the word deflationary. Can you help me a little?

Douglas: Yeah. If you think you're God's creature, then even if your life is miserable and short you have a cosmic importance. When you find out that you're living on speck on the far side of the universe, then even if you live a life that by our standards is rich and exciting and long, you're still facing a lack of that cosmic importance.

Aubrey: The meaning of life. That kind of nonsense. I'm not really into the meaning of life. I'm just a practical guy. I enjoy my life and I'd like to carry on enjoying it and I think that a lot of other people feel the same so I'd like to help them carry on enjoying it too. And that's about as far as my thinking goes on the matter.

Douglas: I kind of expected that that would be what I encountered here, and I don't think that what I'm talking about can easily be summed up just as a question that we ponder, because I think we actually solve those question about the meaning of life and solve them differently through history.

If you asked what the meaning of life was in medieval times, people knew, and it was to serve God's will or something like that. We have different kinds of answers to those questions now. But as our lives change we come up with new answers to those kinds of questions again. The Industrial Revolution changed what we thought the meaning of life was and maybe it didn't matter individually to people, but socially there was a meaning that was being created and that directed people's lives.

But, I'm chattering at you here. Let me skip over some of these questions I have then, the ones based on that one about the meaning of life.

Do you think there are political barriers to your project? And by that I mean, not only are there groups of people who might be opposed and working against you, but also a lack of access to political institutions. If you were to overcome those barriers would you expect your project to have more success more quickly?

Aubrey: Well, sure. There's one really astronomical political barrier which is that, politicians, policy makers, are ultimately tools of the system. The reason they are where they are is because they like being in power, and therefore their motivations for being where they are are very straightforward. They just want to get re-elected.

That means that, public policy does not in any sense lead public opinion, or at least not significantly, it follows public opinion. So at the end of the day this means that it's a complete waste of time for people like myself, or anyone working in radical new technologies, to try to appeal to politicians to actually allocate public funds to this or that thing if they feel there are votes in it. And they'll only feel there are votes in it if they see that there are votes in it when they watch their own televisions and they read their newspapers.

People like myself have to start by influencing public opinion and then public policy will follow suit, will follow along. Then the question is, how does one actually influence public opinion?

41

And the answer, of course, is that one must influence opinion formers. Oprah Winfrey or whatever. But then, of course, the difficulty is that Oprah Winfrey and her ilk got where they are by being very sensitive to what public opinion actually already was, and not trying to shift it too seismically. So one can only do that if one can convince the opinion formers that they are nudging public opinion in a direction that they are going to be praised for in the long run. Which means that one has to convince them that in the scientific community the wind is blowing in that direction. Now, that is, in a nutshell, why I have focused so strongly on the scientific community. They are obviously a very small number of people, but in theory they are smart, and they ought to be able to understand if I'm right. So that's what the campaign has consisted of most of all.

Douglas: Do you think that when you have your first major success in mice that, at that point, it will become a lot easier to gain access to institutional support? And that you'll see a political campaign or movement to speed up the process of this kind of research?

Aubrey: I do. I've always said that there will be an extremely sharp and sudden tipping point in all this. Progress will happen in the laboratory, at our own SENS Research Foundation and elsewhere, and at some point there will be sufficient progress that the very small but, nevertheless, very influential community of senior mainstream gerontologists, will tip to the point of describing that yeah, it's only a matter of time before this all really, really works in humans and not just for mice. And they will be willing to say so on camera, and on stage. That will, I believe, happen relatively suddenly as a result of specific advances that I think are likely to happen within the next five to ten years. And when it does happen everything else will fall like a house of cards. The very next day the opinion formers, the

Oprah Winfreys of this world, are going to be saying, "If it's only a matter of time then maybe we should, you know, make it take less time and save some lives really." And the day after that it'll be impossible to get re-elected unless you have a manifesto commitment to a proper war on aging. You know? To put really serious money behind it. At that point my job will done.

Douglas: If you had that kind of support now, if by some miracle that happened now and there was a government-funded program that was similar to the scale of the program that got us on the moon, how much more quickly do you think we could get to the kind of answers that we need?

Aubrey: Great question. At this point I think we're being held back by roughly a factor of three. If we had infinite money we could go three times faster. Now, when I say infinite money actually I think we would only need about ten times more money to go three times faster. Currently SENS Research Foundation's total annual budget is only five million dollars. So adding one zero to that is still a complete drop in the ocean as compared to medical-research funding in the USA. But what does it mean in terms of the actual amount of time we're losing and the amount of lives we're losing? I don't think it means that, rather than taking twenty or twenty-five years to develop these therapies, which is what I think we could do if money was not a limiting factor, that we'll take sixty to seventy-five years, because as time goes on we will make progress and we will bring more money in and it will speed up. I do think we're looking at at least a ten-year delay. A difference of ten years in how long it's going to take to get these therapies together determined purely on whether or not serious support comes in within the next couple of years.

Douglas: You know, earlier on in our previous conversation I asked you about heart disease and cancer, and I think I

suggested or implied that maybe you could get support from people working on those diseases in particular as you had success.

Do you think that might be a part of what will speed up the process once you start to solve problems that cause one particular disease or another, that you might be able to join hands with people who aren't working specifically on your project?

Aubrey: It turned out to be a pretty complicated question that, actually. On the one hand, for sure, if we develop a therapy that comes of the SENS concept, the damage-repair concept that applies to some particular disease, let's say atherosclerosis, and it really works, then sure, it's going to make big waves and make big money and fund the rest of our work and so on. But, the thing is, in advance of getting it to work, the point where we are at now wanting to push it through, we have to essentially compete with all the other approaches that other researchers are taking against that specific disease. The difficulty is that it's not a level playing field, because when one is focused on only one specific disease one is going to be impressed by very modest advances, even postponement of the progression of atherosclerosis by five years would essentially halve the actual incidence, because people would get other diseases first and die of them. And we don't think that way, we're interested in doing something that's much more dramatic. As such what we're doing is harder to implement, it's at an earlier stage of development.

So, if one goes to someone like the American Heart Association and says we should be funding this research to do this one particular thing they'll say, well hang on. That sounds like a very long shot. Let's do this very much more boring and modest thing because it'll actually give some benefit tomorrow.

Douglas: So if you had all this money, if you had infinite

money, how would you spend it? What is needed right now? Would you just hire more specialists of different kinds to cover the full range of what you're doing all at once, or would you focus more brain power on one particular issue first?

Aubrey: We would not cover one particular issue first. We already cover the bases pretty much. So you probably remember that SENS is this seven-point plan with these seven different types of damage and with each of these we have a particular generic approach for its repair or obviation. The seven-point plan would not change. The way we would spend more money would be partly by doing new projects that fit into this seven-point plan, but mostly by expanding the existing projects. So there are definitely a number of projects we have that could go a lot faster just by the simple expedient of being more parallelized. Being done on a larger scale.

And then, there is work that is essentially stalled because we don't have the money to take it to the next level experimentally. So, for example, just moving from cell cultures into mouse models on a particular disease or a particular aspect of aging. That's clearly a step up eventually, and there are cases where we just don't have that money.

Douglas: That's frustrating.

Let me ask you a question I didn't think of until just now. Who are your allies outside of the medical world? Who do you consider to be allies and where is your support coming from right now?

Aubrey: We have allies all over the place, we just don't have enough of them. A large part of the reason we ended up having our headquarters in Silicon Valley is because Silicon Valley is probably the world's number-one hotbed of visionaries. There are just people, whether it's millionaires or youngsters who want to get involved on the ground, who actually not only understand the value of what we want to do, but they actually want to get involved. Put their money or their time where their mouth is.

Part Three

Outreach, the Media,
the Pro-Aging Trance

Douglas: I'm glad to get a chance to talk to you again and finish this off. Thinking over our conversation so far, I kept returning to this bit where I tried to get you to answer questions about the meaning of life. You frequently probably face this question of whether or not death gives life meaning, and I brought that to you in this sort of convoluted way, and your reluctance to engage in that I understood, but when I thought about it more it seemed to me that you were taking what might be thought of as a logical positivist position about those kinds of questions. I wanted to ask you if you consider yourself a logical positivist.

Aubrey: First of all you're going to have to tell me what a logical positivist is.

Douglas: A logical positivist is someone who thinks that questions about ultimate values, questions that can neither be confirmed tautologically or empirically, are noncognitive. They're just not meaningful statements. But if I have to give you a definition of the term then I'm probably in a terrain where you're not qualified to talk about it very much.

But, I guess the reason why I want to ask you that is because working in the humanities and in the realm of philosophy, publishing books on philosophy of a certain type, these kinds of questions are important to us for strange reasons, and I wanted to ask if you thought it was possible that indefinite life extension would bring challenges to the humanities and bring challenges to our culture that would be unique. If you see that as a possibility. That we're going to have very different kinds of philosophies and art and the rest of it.

Aubrey: Let me do my best to answer that. I certainly believe that the structure of society will change in profound ways when we have indefinite healthy lives, but of course society will change in pretty profound ways as a result of other changes that happen.

Like, you know, the emergence of really comprehensive automation using artificial intelligence, where we don't really have jobs anymore and nothing really costs money anymore. All manner of things like that. I always find it really hard to separate the social and the political from the ethical and the philosophical. It seems to me that the human condition does evolve, does change progressively as the result of technological advances of all kinds. And it's hard to draw a line that says, people are in some fundamental qualitative sense different or living differently than they used to be. I think it's a continuum.

Douglas: It does seem to mean that one small change, I mean it's a drastic change but it's not everything, but one small change in the way that medicine is done could have a very profound effect.

Aubrey: Well, yeah, but those challenges again will be incremental technical changes, like the way that stem cells or the way that surgery is done. I don't really see it, I don't really see a huge difference in terms of that transition, what that transition will look like, from transitions that occur all the time. The progression that develops as a result of new technologies such as keyhole surgery or whatever.

Douglas: I think people might immediately, without there being any real transformation materially in society, when faced with the prospect of an indefinite life... that might have profound psychological effects on people or sociological effects.

Aubrey: If we look at psychological effects, I think a lot of that is overblown. People say, "Oh, wouldn't it be boring living indefinitely? How would we cope? Wouldn't we run out of new things to do?" I think this is crazy.

I think that the way we run our lives today is not based on how long we're going to live. It's not based on how long ago we were born. It's based on relatively short-term considerations. Of course we make long-term decisions based on how long we're going to live that are not psychological, things like which pension plan or health insurance we have. But as psychological things, I just don't see it.

Douglas: I knew a couple who, when they were in their late fifties and early sixties, moved out of their family home, the home where they'd raised their kids, into a smaller apartment. Not just for financial reasons, but because they were projecting into the future where they expected not to be able to handle stairs.

Aubrey: Sure. That's not psychological, that's pragmatic. That's thinking about the options in the future. That's equivalent to health insurance as far as I'm concerned. That's managing one's choices in the context of one's expectations. And as soon as one has a sense of those expectations being different, one will redo those calculations. One will buy cheaper health insurance, or cheaper life insurance, or whatever, because the calculations recommend it. But again it's not a psychological change at all, it's just a pragmatic one.

If you're saying that just that the psychological impact includes things like being happier about the fact that one does not have to look forward to a grim state of health in the future, then sure that's a psychological effect of a kind.

I think you've got a weak definition of the term.

Douglas: I just think that raising people's expectations, elimi- nating the sense that there was a natural order to life and that when you're forty-four you're a different kind of person than you were at twenty-four because of your proximity to the grave,

having those things put aside would change your expectations for your life and how you thought of yourself.

Aubrey: I believe that most of these changes, even today, are not because of one's changing proximity to the grave but because of one's changing proximity to the cradle. One has more abilities, more options available as one goes through life, and of course in due course one gets to the point of having to worry about one's proximity to the grave, but we've already got one's proximity to the cradle aspect and that's not going to change. So, I think it's kind of, it's just easy to see how things would continue more or less as they are, rather than undergoing any fundamental restructuring at the psychological level.

Douglas: One of the things that's frustrating about being middle-aged is that as I get a sense of some sort of mastery of myself in the world, not total mastery by any means, just some basic competence, I realize that I'm on the decline. So, keep working, Aubrey.

Anyhow, let's move on.

You're probably the most famous advocate of indefinite life extension. In the battle to combat age you're the most visible figure I think. Correct me if I'm wrong there.

Aubrey: I probably am, yes.

Douglas: Do you think that it's important for there to be someone in your position, a recognizable personality, associated with this research, with SENS and other research?

Aubrey: I do, yes. I think that this stuff, this stuff needs to be in people's face, in order for people to understand that such a thing can actually happen. People are starting off from the presumption that this is all science fiction, and it has to be beaten over... there has to be someone beating them over the head with the information that the science is moving in that direction.

It's a hard balance, because I don't want it to become a personality cult either. I have to draw a rather fine line between being the personality that people remember, and overshadowing the science.

Douglas: Do you worry that has at times happened, that you've overshadowed the science?

Aubrey: It's different for different audiences isn't it. I think on balance I've probably gotten it about right over the years, but you can never really know.

Douglas: You've been the subject of at least two documentary films. One was produced for Channel 4...

Aubrey: Big ones, that's right. I've also been the subject of lots of much shorter things, but I know the two you're talking about.

Douglas: *Do You Want to Live Forever*, which was on television in Britain, and then this new one which is on Netflix now and is called *The Immortalists*. What did you think about those two films, and I guess maybe the first one *Do You Want to Live Forever*?

Aubrey: Yeah, sure. I saw your comments. You had a rather negative impression or you thought it portrayed me rather negatively. I don't know. There's been a spectrum of opinions there.

There was one little part of that documentary towards the end that was downright fictitious. It was a telephone interview with someone I used to work for in Cambridge who basically became very disaffected with me and gave factually incorrect statements that I didn't know about until afterwards. That was a shame, and of course it did have a negative impact.

But overall I rather felt that the documentary portrayed the whole thing rather positively. I certainly enjoyed very much working with the people who made it. I think they thought it was positive overall. There [are] always constraints in these things in terms of just making the thing popular. They've got to find the money to sell the thing.

On balance my impression was a lot more positive than yours seems to have been.

Douglas: As an interviewer I kind of have to find point of critique. You know, if I just came and said I thought it was great then there wouldn't be as much talk. I have to find an oppositional point, but I agree it was certainly not a black-and-white issue.

I watched that film and was fascinated by what you were doing and found you to be a charismatic character in the film. That's definitely the up side to it. The down side to it is that the narrative of the lone genius puts you in a marginal position, and also I found that the focus kept shifting from the science to the personal in ways I wasn't comfortable with, just intellectually. I didn't like it. I thought it was cheap often. There was a conversation they recorded between you and a molecular biologist or a geneticist. I would have loved it if they had just stayed on that conversation for an hour or something. Let me hear you guys actually talk about this stuff, but it switched tracks from how feasible, in a typical way, how feasible the project was, to questioning your motivations and whether or not you had children and that kind of thing.

Aubrey: I agree. That kind of thing...

Again, I feel things like this... if I didn't have anything about myself that was worth talking about then they probably wouldn't have made the documentary at all and that would have probably been less good for the mission. So that's part of what I'm saying about the balance between having... being somewhat memorable.

Douglas: That's something about the form of the television documentary is that they have to personalize every story. Although...

Aubrey: The big profiles that have been done on me in the print media, the same applies really. They have the same kind of constraints, the same kind of reasons to have that mixture. To perhaps have more of the personality side than I would ideally wish.

Douglas: They don't actually do that to everyone. There are scientists whose discoveries are deemed to be significant enough that they do not need to be personalized.

Aubrey: But those scientist don't have ninety minutes made about them. Those scientists get in the news for ten minutes once in their career. So, I think it's important for this... I think it's a good thing that I've become something of a media fixture. It's sometimes surprising you know. I totally thought ten years ago that people would get pretty bored of me pretty soon, but it doesn't seem to have happened.

Douglas: One thing I didn't ask and I want to find out is how did you go through the process of changing your career from being a computer scientist to working in gerontology and combating aging? How quickly did you realize that you wanted to be both someone who was spearheading a scientific inquiry and a kind of figurehead and spokesperson?

Aubrey: How I made the transition. I was just in an extraordinarily fortunate situation. So, I started out working in artificial-intelligence research. I had, during the late second half of the '80s, I had the great good fortune to be teaming up with a guy who had inspired the project originally, the project that I was working on, but who also had enough marketable programming skills, much more than I did actually, to be able to pay the bills for the two of us. So I was basically a full-time researcher in a two-man company. That money eventually ran out around 1991 or so, and I had to actually have, for a grim six or eight months, where I had to have a proper job, writing code that would actually work. It was no fun at all. But, that was in 1992. I'd met my wife in 1990 and she of course, as you've seen, is a lifelong biologist. By the time we'd been together a couple of years, I knew a lot of biology, especially fruit-fly genetics which is her field. And then a job turned up, this bioinformatics position at the University of Cambridge which was a new project being co-led by the same person whose lab my wife was working in, and he offered me this job.

Initially I thought this was an idiotic idea because I thought it was going to be really boring, but Adelaide, my wife, pointed out to me that it would also be really undemanding, and it would give me a lot of free time, with the result that I would be able to revive my artificial-intelligence research. I quite rapidly realized that she was absolutely right so I took the job.

Sure enough, after an initial period of, you know, setup I guess… for about a year, it did indeed turn out to be really undemanding and I did indeed start thinking in terms of starting new artificial-intelligence projects. So that was in 1994.

But, it was around that time that it was beginning to sink in that not only Adelaide, but also every other biologist I was meeting, was actually completely crazy when it came to aging. They didn't understand that it was an important or interesting problem, and they were not working on it. And I eventually came to the conclusion that I needed to switch fields because, there were various reasons why I felt that I had a good chance of making a respectable contribution to the field of gerontology, in terms of hastening the defeat of aging. I just thought I had the right kind of talents, and I was in a position to do so. Because the research I was doing in artificial intelligence was being done entirely in my spare time, of which I was able to carve out quite a lot. I was just re-purposing my spare time and there was no risk involved in that.

Douglas: Once you started to do that, to re-purpose your spare time and do the research, when did you realize that a maintenance approach to combating aging was the way to go? Maybe you knew that earlier?

Aubrey: No, I didn't know that. You had another part to your previous question, of course, which was when did I become aware…

Douglas: Right, I want to get back to that because I want to dig in a little bit more about the process of change in career and a little bit on what it took for you to formulate this approach.

Aubrey: Sure, so the maintenance approach… no, that certainly was not apparent to me from the beginning. It was not apparent to anybody. I went into gerontology as a novice, not knowing anything about the field except the general biology that I'd learned from my wife over the dinner table, and so I spent five and a half years, I'm going to say starting in 1995, essentially learning. You know. Going to a lot of conferences because my undemanding bioinformatics job was giving me a nice salary and I could afford to pay my way to conferences, you know getting to know the people, getting to know a lot of science. I was publishing stuff, I was making contributions during that period, but they were harmless contributions. I was publishing papers that would, you know, give new explanations for ostensibly paradoxical results and things like that.

And that was all very fine, but basically what I was doing was absorbing information, turning things over in my mind, and waiting essentially for the eureka moment. Waiting to come up with an idea that hadn't been had and that was more promising. And that's what happened in the summer of 2000. I had this big revelation in Los Angeles at this two-day workshop that I'd been invited to participate in, and I suddenly saw that everyone had rejected this concept. That everyone was going for slowing down the accumulation of damage, the creation of damage, and there were only isolated examples where people were thinking at all in terms of repairing damage. And I realized that, actually the concept of repairing damage could be made much more comprehensive. The way I did it was by incorporating, by bringing in, a lot of science that gerontologists had never even thought about or heard about, stuff that I'd been able to discover just because I had been going about my explorations in an extremely adventurous way. I'd been going to a very diverse range of conferences, reading a very diverse range of scientific literature, and so on. I brought in all these new ideas and put them together into a coherent framework that was this seven-point plan. It just hung together and I realized, my God, this actually could work. We could actually repair all the relevant, all the important damage.

And of course it took years after that for the concept of damage, for comprehensive damage repair, to get to any kind of level of orthodoxy the way it is now. Because there was so much that gerontologists, that my colleagues in the field, had never even heard of.

Douglas: When you came upon this idea and you realized that the reason you were able to think of it was because you were not as mired in the everyday thicket of detail that other gerontologists are but had a more comprehensive view, did you realize at that point that this idea would need a spokesperson,

that it was not going to be picked up easily by the established scientific or medical community, or did that come later?

Aubrey: Kind of, kind of... I knew that the established bio-gerontologist community was the most important audience. If they decided I was right then they would start saying I was right to journalists and opinion formers, and once opinion formers started to believe that there was a new idea that had a lot of promise then, the whole house of cards collapses at once. Basically the public starts thinking that, and then policy makers start thinking that, and then my job is done.

But, I also realized that this is kind of circular. The gerontologists were not going to say this if they think the initial consequence is going to be that the work they're already doing, the work they're already experts at, is going to be de-prioritized. They're going to see it as an attack on their established research programs, so they're going to be resistant. And of course I'm not the first person to have that insight, people were saying for an awfully long time that science advances funeral by funeral, and this is why.

Essentially I realized that I did need to appeal to everybody, not just to the group working on the biology of aging, and I went on tour.

And so when I started coming to the attention of the futurist community, people who are interested in this, in radical life extension, and in artificial intelligence, and nanotechnology, and so on... I was very happy about that, and I enthusiastically went and made talks in those communities. We're talking about 2002, that kind of period.

Then it kind of spiraled. People started sending invitations to more high-profile things, of course that ended up with me being invited to speak at TED in 2006. Actually I gave my first TED talk in 2005. And you can't do much better than that for exposure to people who can make a difference. That was the main source of our initial boost of funding.

So yeah, I realized from the beginning that I had to do this.

Douglas: Did you find that doing the public speaking and being a public advocate was a unique kind of challenge? Did you already have any background in that kind of work, or did it just come naturally to you?

Aubrey: That's a great question. In a sense it came naturally to me. I've always known that I'm reasonably charismatic, and determined. I knew I had very good material as well. I knew that I had the potential to tell a good story and to be persuasive. On the other hand, no, I did not have any training in public speaking or even... I never even had a teaching position at the university, for example. So, at the beginning I really wasn't very good at it. I had an enormous difficulty stopping myself from speaking too fast, for example.

But, basically I always felt I could make a reasonable job of it. Of course I got progressively better as the years have gone by.

Douglas: Did you get some help once you started or did you record yourself, take a look at it, and try to adjust your behavior that way?

Aubrey: A bit of both. Of course, other people would offer encouragement or advice and so on, but yeah I used to actually rehearse my talks.

Douglas: Well, back to the films. I have a question that I didn't get to raise before. Maybe you'll be able to answer or at least express an opinion about it.

Do you think that there is something in the culture now that acts as a conservative force to stop people thinking not just about what you are researching, but that stops people thinking

in an open way, and that maybe the way that things are personalized might have something to do with it?

I noticed in the film *Do You Want to Live Forever*, they would frequently, not just a couple of times, frequently start with a scientific question, or at least a question that had to do with logic, and move to an answer which was pretty much exclusively personal. So they asked you if you thought people would get more creative as they got older after a successful medical intervention that could maintain the brain and maintain the body, and you gave an opinion on that. And they turn around to get a second opinion by asking an entirely different question to Freedman Dyson.

And he says, "I think that if people from the 17th century were still alive they'd be a terribly conservative force and they wouldn't be creative." It's really not the same question that's being asked.

Do you think that kind of thing happens a lot?

Aubrey: I think the raising of the questions that I get and that other people get is part of the issue, but really it's all a package. Everyone's got an agenda. The filmmaker wants to slant the questions, and the answers for that matter, in a manner that tells a story that they want to tell. That they think is going to sell. That they're interested in. And similarly I or Freeman... the answers that we give [are] only loosely determined by the questions we get. I think that's kind of okay, because it kind of reveals not only what people think but what people want other people to think.

I know why most people have these absurd, knee-jerk, negative vibes about what a post-aging world is going to be like, whether it's about cognitive ossification as in the example you're talking about, or whether it's overpopulation, or dictators living forever, or anything. I know that, you know, as you've seen, I have this phrase the "Pro-Aging Trance" where people have to get into this stance just to put it out of their minds. But, if you're asking really why do interviewers and interviewees talk this way, it's in the nature of the media. You're trying to promote your point of view.

Douglas: I guess, when you're trying to answer scientific questions, if you approach questions the way we do in the media, there would be very little progress. If you ask "Does this gene do X?" and your answer had something to do with blood or something else, then—

Aubrey: I hate to break it to you, Doug, but the fact is that problem does indeed exist in science.

Douglas: Oh, no...

Aubrey: People do the science that they think... Most scientists are ultimately careerists. They may have been idealists at the beginning of their careers but they lose their ideals very quickly under the tyranny of system. The fact of having to bloody, you know, get their next grant funded. Get their next promotion. Get their PHD students and postdocs in a position to get promoted themselves, and so on...

If you get a senior scientist wickedly drunk and you ask them to give you a straight answer with regard to whether they're actually doing what they'd like to do, whether they're doing the science that they would do if they had unlimited funds that were completely secure and under their own control indefinitely, then they will tell you no way. They will tell you that they are compromising all the time, in terms of what they are actually choosing to do.

Douglas: Does that happen at SENS?

Aubrey: No. The reason that SENS exists is precisely because we need such compromise not to happen. We go out and get money and we spend it the way we think it needs to be spent.

Douglas: One last question about the films and all of that, and this is out of context and it's a good example of me not letting you and the logic of this conversation direct me but having my own agenda, but I wouldn't be able to... I feel I need to ask this question. I could certainly live with myself if I didn't, but I want to ask it.

In the second film that we haven't talked about very much, the film *The Immortalists*, which is much more sympathetic. It too focuses on your personal life I think in ways that are much less counterproductive, but which are questionable at times.

I just have to ask you, what was your thinking when you allowed them to document what I'll call the "naked picnic scene"?

Aubrey: A lot of people have asked me that, including my outreach people. I'm just not very smart, I guess. You know. I...

I'm a very unconventional guy in a lot of ways, some of which came out in the film, some of which didn't, and I don't really see how people are going to see me.

Douglas: Do you want to go on? It sounds like there is a pregnant pause building here.

Aubrey: No. That's really all there is to say. I don't really have anything more that's left over on that.

Douglas: Okay. So you weren't trying to make your own cultural statement there or advocate for more liberated sexuality, or a more liberated life. It wasn't a political statement.

Aubrey: No. It wasn't my idea. You know, the filmmakers spent a long time with me, same as the filmmakers for the previous film spent a long time with me, and they knew all about my life, and they had their own idea about what aspect of it that they wanted to include and they would make requests, and I would generally say sure.

Douglas: I was going to ask you about George Monbiot who is associated with the left and has kind of critiqued your project in ways that I thought were typically unfair and not very thoughtful... I guess what I want to ask you is where do you find the most resistance? Do you find the left, or people who are supposedly on the liberal side, are more likely or less likely to be resistant to you?

Aubrey: I haven't really seen much of a difference. The only political grouping that one would say is actually different from most is libertarians, who are disproportionately among our supporters, but I don't think your typical libertarian would view themselves as being particularly left or particularly right.

Douglas: I'll tell you this, the left that I'm associated with would consider libertarians to be, American libertarians, to be on the right. I wouldn't entirely disagree with them, but not entirely agree either. But from so-called progressives, people who define themselves as on the left, you find that there are just as many for as against you is usually the case.

Aubrey: Yes.

**Douglas: Okay, so let's talk about the pro-aging trance a little bit more.
Do you think the pro-aging trance has diminished?**

Aubrey: It's only diminished very slightly. It's still enormously the case that we get people, first of all immediately coming up with the standard knee-jerk reaction against the concept of a post-aging world, whether it's feasibility or it's desirability, and second of all being very uninterested in the actual answers that show them that they're wrong. So, yeah there are... there are signs of movement, but those are not signs within the overall general public. You know...

It's become a more acceptable topic of conversation than it used to be, but really that topic... that's because people see, they see more of it in the media, they see it being treated more sympathetically in the media. I don't think it really demonstrates a change in people's inherent attitudes. It's more a case that people would be embarrassed to be as negative and as dismissive as they used to be.

Douglas: Well I found as I raised the subject of this interview on social media that I got the peculiar but yet well-established response I've seen so many times. Just when I asked the question about what people think of your project. I got from people who consider themselves radical, very conservative answers. Some of them almost religious, but the main response was this rejection of life. This feeling "Oh, who really wants this to go on this long?"

Do you feel that the pro-aging trance is a reflection of people's depression?

Aubrey: Depression. Well depression is an interesting word to use. Fatalism, perhaps, is better. I've described the pro-aging trance very explicitly as a coping strategy, a way of avoiding the psychological trauma of hoping for something that might or might not come to pass in time. That's really what it comes down to. And yeah, you can call it depression, you can call it being down-trodden.

Douglas: There is this parable written by Nick Bostrom. It's called "The Fable of the Dragon Tyrant," and you think this a pretty accurate fable. It may not be great literature, but in it people come to accept life with a mighty dragon, a dragon who can't be killed. You know the story.

It demands human flesh and human sacrifice, and history rolls along and society adapts. They develop even sciences to make it easier to offer up human sacrifices to the great dragon, programs to facilitate those other programs, and there is a whole economy of this.

Where are we in this parable and are we at the point in the story where people recognize the need to dismantle all these different apparatuses and make an effort to kill the dragon?

Aubrey: We're quite a lot further away than that. It's at the very early stage.

It's so early. You know, we've got incremental progress in the laboratory. Look at the situation with the SENS Research Foundation's funding. We got Peter Thiel for one just as soon as I came to the attention of anybody. I was certain back then that things would progress at a smooth accelerating rate, and in fact it took four more years for Jason Hope, the IT entrepreneur from Arizona, to come in at the same kind of level, a few hundred thousand a year or more, up to half a million. And that's it, you know. We have still not got a significant stream of really high net-worth people coming in, so you've got to ask why. How long is it going to stay that way?

Honestly, you know I'm an optimist. I've worked really hard to make this happen, and I keep trying to believe that tomorrow and tomorrow it'll actually happen. But, honestly we don't know. I really think the pro-aging trance is alive and well at the moment.

Douglas: Do you think that the problem is that most people don't view this project as desirable?

Aubrey: It depends on what you mean by view. I mean, as I say, it's a trance, right? It's not a rational opinion.

Douglas: That's what I mean. Is the pro-aging trance right now… [are] most of the objections you're going to get from people who have the resources to help going to take the form of a moral argument? Do they say, "No, I don't want to overcome aging"?

Aubrey: Every high net-worth individual is different, but I certainly think that among the more visionary end of the high net-worth spectrum, the people I end up talking to, the people who I meet at TED for example, the idea that this is undesirable is not a particularly high bar. I think that by and large those people are not susceptible to that kind of "logic." They do, however, have a different problem. A lot of these people, and I can tell you this from some of these people who have actually been explicit about this, the main reason they're not giving us money is because their spouses don't want us to. Because their spouses are not as visionary as they are.

In other words, their objections really are about whether it's desirable. If we factor that out, then the next question is, is the whole enterprise feasible? Do we have a plan that actually hangs together? And of course these people don't know, they're not biologists. They have to identify somehow to actually, in some way, trust. And of course they don't know who to trust either. So, it's again rather circular. They end up trusting the wrong people.

If you get past that and they tell themselves that this does actually hang together well enough, then the question is are we the right team? Is this something that should be done in a nonprofit context, by a charity such as SENS? A lot of these people just like to think that way, because they got to be high net-worth individuals by making money. They believe in the power of the market and all that. I think that could be a large part of why the Google twins ended up never giving us any money, and eventually giving a large amount of money to a spin-out company called Calico, which may or may not contribute to the overall mission in the long run. Everyone's different.

Douglas: What are the most hopeful signs that occurred recently? Where should people who are wanting to be optimistic look to get excited?

Aubrey: Well obviously we're doing the right stuff. We know that we're doing the right stuff. We spend a lot of time making sure that we're doing the right stuff, so I'd say look at our website.

Douglas: The last time I spoke to you you'd just published a paper a day earlier, and I think I saw today on my Facebook an alert about another new development. Are these things happening rather regularly where you're making a significant advance every month? How is the progress going?

Aubrey: That's actually a pretty hard question as well. It depends on what you mean by advance. You could measure it at the level of publications. Or it could exist at the level of stuff I know about that's going on internally.

I'm really excited, because I see all of these things happening. It's easy for me to stay excited and to see progress constantly. But the progress that's been of a sufficient magnitude in terms of the increment from where we were before to actually get a publication like that one you're mentioning, that happens fairly rarely. Yes, the frequency is increasing, but it still needs to increase a lot more.

Douglas: As you've gone along have you won converts within the scientific community? I mean real converts. People who

started out opposing you, maybe publically, who have come around to at least support your research if not participate in it?

Aubrey: Absolutely. Lots of them.

Ten years ago, as you know, we had a lot of very public opposition. Opposition that was actually, more or less, engineered by me. Because it was happening already, but it was happening off the record. That was very hard to respond to, and I smoked out my more vocal detractors and got them so angry that they actually started saying things in print, and that allowed me to rebut the critiques.

But yeah, this was very widespread back then. Of course most of the movement has been not all the way, there are people who have gone from being vocal detractors to being on the fence, or they've gone from being on the fence to being vocal supporters. You get the idea.

Absolutely, we certainly wouldn't be able to have the SENS advisory board that we have if there had not been that process of bringing people on board.

Douglas: Can you think of something that was the most convincing to people within the scientific community who opposed you? Was there a moment? Was it the publication in the *Technology Review* where they couldn't discredit your ideas as unscientific, or was there any particular argument that seemed to be the most effective with people that moved them onto the fence or onto your side?

Aubrey: I would not say there was any particular argument, no. I think it was the overall climate of the argument. The fact that when people saw the actual exchanges they realized that they lacked a lot of information. They had come to an opinion based on a gut feeling about the plausibility of what I was saying and that they had not done their homework. When they saw people actually laying out their criticisms of SENS, and saw those criticisms rebutted on the basis of published information, actual experimental work that should have been already known to the people who were criticizing in the first place, but wasn't known to them because they hadn't taken the trouble to read my papers, or read the work that I was citing, then it became obvious who was being unscientific and who wasn't.

Contemporary culture has eliminated both the concept of the public and the figure of the intellectual. Former public spaces – both physical and cultural – are now either derelict or colonized by advertising. A cretinous anti-intellectualism presides, cheerled by expensively educated hacks in the pay of multinational corporations who reassure their bored readers that there is no need to rouse themselves from their interpassive stupor. The informal censorship internalized and propagated by the cultural workers of late capitalism generates a banal conformity that the propaganda chiefs of Stalinism could only ever have dreamt of imposing. Zer0 Books knows that another kind of discourse – intellectual without being academic, popular without being populist – is not only possible: it is already flourishing, in the regions beyond the striplit malls of so-called mass media and the neurotically bureaucratic halls of the academy. Zer0 is committed to the idea of publishing as a making public of the intellectual. It is convinced that in the unthinking, blandly consensual culture in which we live, critical and engaged theoretical reflection is more important than ever before.